H.E.A.L.T.H.
It's Not Rocket
Science
(My Journey to a Healthier Me)

Bridget McCray

DEDICATION

This is dedicated to my husband, Joel. Thank you for the endless support and encouragement you give, as well as for continuing to challenge me to think outside of the box. I could not imagine life without you, Babe. I love you.

What People Are Saying …

"I love Bridget's honest and straightforward approach about how to reclaim your health. Her delivery is humorous and oh so relatable. Her story is like so many of ours. But, the compassion that she has shown herself is the same compassion that she shows her clients each and every day. She gives encouragement, and her 'take it one step at a time' approach keeps you motivated to stay the course of your journey."

Carla Henslee
Owner, Premier Yoga &
Fitness
www.premieryogafit.com

"Bridget received a wake up call from a pretty serious health concern. She could have written it off or taken a long path to wellness with prescribed medication. However, she chose the path of H.E.A.L.T.H. We, as a family, are proud of her for embracing this lifestyle change. Her story of spiritual, mental, and physical transformation is encouraging, practical, and inspiring. You will be blessed by this book, and I hope you will be inspired to embrace H.E.A.L.T.H. as a new lifestyle."

Joel McCray
Composer, Producer
Owner, Fast Track Records
www.joelmccray.com
www.fasttrackrecords.com

"Bridget's authenticity and transparency in her own health journey encourages the reader to start NOW, not later, even if a small step, towards a healthier lifestyle. Her positive disposition shines throughout the chapters and makes it super easy for the busiest of us to apply her suggestions. She comes along side the reader and whispers thought provoking questions to encourage, inform and coach us on our very own personal health journey. Excellent read!"

Barbara Schermerhorn
Certified Public Accountant
www.paperdoll.me

"Bridget's journey to better health continues to inspire me daily. Her dedication to feel better and live a long, healthy, and fulfilled life for not only herself, but for her family also, is admirable. As she continues her journey, I enjoy observing the adjustments to her eating habits, exercise, and rest to best fit her needs. She went from being a novice individual that had little experience with exercise and limited knowledge about nutrition to an individual who is a group fitness instructor, as well as a personal trainer. She also encourages others to listen to their bodies and make adjustments in both exercise and nutrition. Her positive outlook gives inspiration to others around her, as well as myself. She has made me have many 'aha' moments. I am proud to call her friend, and I know her journey will inspire and encourage others."

Veronica Valadez
Registered Nurse

"Our God is an Awesome God! It has absolutely been an honor to watch Mrs. McCray become Isaiah 58, 'God's Walking Billboard!' When Bridget and I first started this journey, she felt like God was calling her to be a model. Little did she know God had His picture in mind for what that model would look like for Kingdom expansion. Well, she has become that model that our Lord has called her to be. This book, the first of many, will be used as a guideline to help others become the model that God is calling all of us to be, 'God's Walking Billboard!'"

Dr. Japonica Walker
Doctor of Naturopathy
Essence of Excellence
www.japonicawalker.com

Bridget McCray

CONTENTS

Acknowledgments

Introduction   1

1 **H**ave a Plan   3

2 **E**at & Exercise with Purpose   9

3 **A**lter Your Thinking   19

4 **L**eave Behind Old Habits   29

5 **T**eam Up   37

6 **H**ave Faith   43

   Worksheets   55

   Disclaimer   65

Bridget McCray

ACKNOWLEDGMENTS

I would like to express my appreciation to:

My husband of almost 19 years, Joel, for his continued love, encouragement, and support: He is my friend, my confidant, and the love of my life. As the earthly head of our home, he leads with wisdom, with laughter, and with strength. I cannot express adequately in words how grateful I am to have him in my life as husband and as father to our children.

My children, Nicholas and Jada, who bring immense joy to my life: I never knew that being a mother would be something that I would so treasure. They are reminders of the importance of my change in lifestyle, as it pertains to my health. They are the next generation and are truly blessings.

My parents, Dianne Reimonenq and Roland Doucette, Sr., as well as my second mom, Patricia Doucette, for their constant support over the years: Through "thick and thin," they have shown unconditional love, which I cherish.

My "mom-in-love," Ruby McCray, for her prayers and encouragement for my family and me: She is the one who initially challenged me, through her own lifestyle, to begin taking a closer look at what I was eating and to start making better choices.

My friend, Dr. Japonica Walker, N.D., for the practical advice she has provided, starting with a perceived random encounter almost four years ago: The tools, with which she has equipped me, have been pivotal in the transformation of my health. Her wisdom has been invaluable.

My mentor, Tom Pryor, for graciously sharing his expertise without reservation: He has not only been a business mentor, but also a friend to both my husband and me. He has challenged us to think differently about finances and entrepreneurship. His insight has been priceless.

My friend, Terri Cooper, for speaking words of affirmation regarding the writing of this book: She had no idea at the time that I had already been inspired to do this months earlier, yet sadly, I had been procrastinating. Unbeknownst to her, it was through her words that I was moved with a sense of urgency to finish what I'd started.

My family members and friends, as well as fellow fitness instructors, who have motivated me and cheered me on as I have walked this journey: Your support has been a blessing.

Lastly, and most importantly, I would like to thank my Father in Heaven for the gift of His Son, my Savior and my Lord, Jesus Christ, by the power of His Holy Spirit. Through His death, burial, and resurrection from the dead, I have new and everlasting life. It is under His inspiration that I have the privilege to write this book in an effort to be a blessing to others in a practical way.

INTRODUCTION

"Better late than never" is certainly a familiar saying, and I believe it adequately describes the start of my journey to better health. You see, my "Aha!" moment did not happen until I was in my mid-forties.

Why in the world did I not make a change sooner?? What was I thinking?? There was no shortage of information that could have helped me. Is it possible that, secretly, I did not really want to know the truth? Though not everything on the web is accurate, of course, I could have done some research on the internet and used common sense to discern the good from the bad.

Speaking of discernment, how about those commercials promising things along the lines of being able to "lose 40 pounds and 20 inches in one week" if you'll just take this pill, or "exercise for only five minutes a day"? Seriously?? It's all about a "quick fix"?? What happens after the weight and inches are lost so quickly, but the person's habits have not changed? Hmmm… You guessed it: most likely he or she will not only gain back what was lost, but will also gain even more.

Though weight was never my concern, I felt as if the promotion of the idea by some advertisers that lasting change could happen "overnight" is so very tempting. Who wouldn't want to have the "magic pill" to make everything better and quickly, right? However, this idea is a farce. There are no lasting results in "quick fixes." Not withstanding a miracle (and yes, I believe they still occur), real change comes through the choices we make daily.

I decided that instead of beating myself up for taking so long to "get it", I would choose to be grateful I did finally get it. When I started to actually practice the notion that real change happens through my daily decisions, this is when transformation began. Little did I know at the time that as the appearance of my physical body improved, others were noticing, then started asking questions. That's when I realized my journey was not just about me.

In the pages of this book, I will be sharing about practical things I have experienced in the turnaround of my own health. **It is important to note that in no way is this information intended to serve as medical advice**; it is simply my personal story. Should you choose to embark upon a journey to better your health, **please consult with a physician before doing so**.

My prayer and hope is that each one reading about my personal journey to improved health would not only be encouraged, but also motivated to action, experiencing his or her own positive transformation, in order to fulfill his or her destiny without health issues as hindrances.

1 HAVE A PLAN

Is your schedule flat-out busy? Are you an entrepreneur? Do you work for an employer, such as a school district, a hospital, a corporation, or a non-profit organization? Are you a stay-at-home mom? Whether or not you have children, is your daily agenda full of things to do? Can you relate to any of the following:

- You realize that you're carrying more weight than you'd prefer.
- You would like to get healthier but don't really know where or how to begin.
- Your lifestyle has become sedentary.
- You've tried to take better care of yourself in the past, but it seemed that your efforts resulted in only short-term successes, followed by frustration, which led to emotional eating and less physical activity, like a vicious cycle.
- You feel like there aren't enough hours in a day to do all that you need to do.

If any of these scenarios resonate with you, I hope you will continue to read, as I share how I came to develop a plan for success in my journey to better overall health by using small, attainable goals to:

- Slowly improve my eating habits
- Start drinking a sufficient amount of water daily
- Make regular exercise a part of my life

The Wake-up Call

In February 2012, I had a "wake up call". One day, my husband mentioned that he could hear my breathing from across the room. I had not just finished anything strenuous, so this was certainly not normal. We discovered that my resting heart rate (RHR) was 100 beats per minute (bpm).

Also, after a recent headache, he suggested that I check my blood pressure. It had always been fine when I went to the doctor. However, this time, at the young age of 45, my blood pressure was hardly fine; it was 188/100. Whoa!

Between the RHR and blood pressure readings, it was crystal clear that the time to make some changes had come! My husband said, "WE are going to start walking." He was already physically fit, having been a star athlete in high school and in college, and he was still in great shape; yet, he felt that it was important to help me by literally walking by my side. I was (and still am) so grateful for that.

Due to modifications in his schedule, he could no

longer walk with me consistently. Not long after that, I joined a gym, because I did not feel comfortable walking alone outside. I'd seen great improvement in my RHR after walking with my husband. My heart rate had dropped from 100 bpm to 70 bpm in roughly five months. This was progress.

However, I felt a sense of disappointment that my blood pressure had not decreased to the same degree that my RHR had. After a few months at the gym, my pressure still had not been reduced much. I even allowed a doctor to prescribe medication for me, and I took that for a short time. Consequently, after he adjusted the dosage a couple of times, and to no avail, his nurse practitioner told me that some people have to take blood pressure medicine for the rest of their lives.

I do not recall the doctor or the nurse practitioner mentioning anything about how I could incorporate exercise and/or make dietary changes in an effort to lower my blood pressure. This was alarming to me! In that moment, I decided I would NOT resign myself to the idea that I would be required to take pharmaceutical drugs for the rest of my life. Personally, I did not want to live my life being a slave to medication.

I realized that there was no time like the present. I could not wait any longer to start taking care of myself, for tomorrow is not promised to any of us. I

remembered that I only have one body on this earth, so it would behoove me to care for it well. I reminded myself that I was created to accomplish great things for God's glory. It would be wonderful to be able to achieve them without having to worry about my health.

I didn't know exactly how to go about integrating necessary changes, but I knew that with all God has provided, be it fruits and vegetables, connections to people, or access to information via the internet, there had to be a way to get healthier without medication. But...how? Where would I even start in order to begin seeing major improvements? I needed a workable plan.

Roughly two years later, I saw a lady, whom I'd met years ago, while I was at the gym. We were next to each other on cardio machines and were having what I thought was a casual conversation; yet, it was a divine appointment, indeed. I truly believe that this was by the grace of God.

As I spoke of the frustration I was feeling, to the point that I'd almost discontinued my gym membership, she told me that the problem was with my diet. Unbeknownst to me at the time, she was a certified personal trainer. I was also unaware that at the time when we became reacquainted, she was studying to become a Doctor of Naturopathy. She is Dr. Japonica Walker, N.D. To say that she has been a Godsend is an understatement! She felt that God told her to help me, and that she did! She shared practical tools to help me take charge of my health.

What she did **not** do was give me a rigid plan to follow. She explained that I might not like to eat the same things that she does, which made perfect sense. She told me something very important to remember during my journey: Make the process look like me. The journey to a healthier lifestyle is not "one size fits all". If we find what works for us, we are much more likely to stick with it.

I recall her asking me to record everything I ate for three days, so that she could review it. I had a pretty good idea about a couple of areas needing improvement, and she confirmed those.

In all honesty, I was a little bit nervous at first. I mean, certainly I knew I would need to make some dietary changes if I expected to see more improvement in my health. However, in my mind, that would be monumental, a major overhaul. The initial thought of that was downright scary to me; that is, until she encouraged me to make one small change at a time. That way, it wouldn't seem overwhelming. This was wise advice.

Having a plan with small, attainable goals is

something that Dr. Walker helped me to understand is critical to success in improving my health. This can be especially useful if the plan is a written one.

Valuing small victories is important. One does not reach the top of a mountain with one giant leap. Right? It happens one small step at a time. (I've had to remind myself of this many a time.) The same idea applies in trying to better one's health. Perfection is not required, but consistency is.

Takeaway: When we make a plan with small, attainable goals, we can see success if we follow through on that plan with consistency.

Action: Identify three <u>specific</u> things that you would like to change regarding the current state of your health.

(1) _____

(2) _____

(3) _____

Notes:

_____

_____

_____

2 **E**AT & EXERCISE WITH PURPOSE

I knew that I needed to do better regarding my sugar intake and my sodium intake, as I figured I was consuming far more than I should have been. Dr. Walker suggested that I look at the foods I was already eating and try to find healthier options for those, one at a time; so, I did. If I recall correctly, it was the first time in my life that I was actually reading the nutrition labels on products I was buying. This was definitely an eye-opening experience!

Baby Steps

A few areas where I first made changes were with peanut butter, turkey bacon, and milk. I've enjoyed peanut butter for as long as I can remember. I would eat it by the tablespoon right from the jar. (Don't laugh. ☺) Yet, I was willing to try something else, something similar.

Though I'd always liked peanuts, I had never really been a fan of almonds; however, I was open to getting out of my comfort zone with almond butter as a possible alternative to peanut butter. I looked at the contents on the labels of both jars and noticed that there was a significant difference in the amount of sodium in the two nut butters. The brand of peanut butter that I'd been eating contained twice as much sodium (and sugar) as the almond butter did. It seemed like that would be an easy change to make. I found that I actually liked the almond butter and have eaten it almost daily since then. I do still have a spoonful of peanut butter, but only on occasion.

My family and I had been eating turkey bacon for a few years, so I sought out to find healthier options for it. I discovered that there are lower sodium options, as well as something called "uncured" turkey bacon. At the time, I was unfamiliar with this term. I learned that it is less processed than regular turkey bacon. I was able to compare packages to determine which choice was best for my family overall.

No! Not That!

Milk…ah…milk! My all-time favorite drink, from childhood to adulthood! I could have it for breakfast, lunch, and dinner. Milk was filling and tasted really good to me, especially if I added flavored powders or syrups. Mmmm!! It really hadn't occurred to me that milk could be a contributing factor to the severe acne with which I'd suffered for so long. Certainly, how could something that I was taught would build strong bones possibly not be good for my body??

Dr. Walker suggested that I consider having a food allergy test done, in order to determine if there was something in my diet to which my body was having a negative reaction. Doing so had never crossed my mind. When I thought of food allergies in the past, I envisioned someone breaking out in hives, or having a swelling of the tongue, neither of which I'd ever personally experienced.

After having an allergy test done, the results indicated that dairy products are ones I should only consume sparingly. What?? In my mind, that would surely be something extremely difficult to do, but I did…one choice at a time, one day at a time.

I tried almond milk and liked it, especially chocolate almond milk; however, almond milk from the store has almost no protein. (I'd learned about the necessity of protein for building and repairing muscle tissue, which was important to know, since I'd started lifting weights.) In addition, store-bought chocolate almond milk has lots of sugar; so, I knew I'd have to increase my protein intake through other foods, as well as monitor my overall sugar intake daily. There is unsweetened almond milk, but my brain was <u>not</u> on board with that at first. I had to slowly work my way into it. This was a process, but I did eventually "catch the vision".

Sweat It Out

As an adult, exercise was a dirty word to me. Who wants to get all sweaty?? I know I didn't…well, not initially. I only saw it as something that teachers and coaches said should be done. I don't remember seeing many adults exercising when I was growing up. Since I didn't see many grown-ups doing it, surely that meant it wasn't important. Didn't it? (I'd made all kinds of excuses.)

It wasn't until I made the decision that I was going to exercise, and do so consistently, that I began to see change. This was definitely not normal for me, but one day at a time, it was becoming my "new norm". Not only was I getting stronger, but my physique also began to reflect it, especially when I started to incorporate resistance training (lifting weights). In addition, my stamina was improving, and so was my balance and flexibility. After experiencing those positive changes, I realized the process was well worth the sweat!

When I began exercising regularly, I would wear a heart rate monitor, mostly because I thought it looked cool initially. (Did I just say that??) The monitor also counted calories, so I'd know how many I burned when I'd workout. Once I was finished, I would take a picture of the monitor, displaying my heart rate and the number of calories I'd expended, then post the photo on social media with the aim of encouraging others to get up and get moving.

When one is a parent, daily life can surely require stamina. As we get "younger", as my mom-in-love says, balance, muscular strength, and flexibility are all important, too. Why? Wouldn't you love to be able to pick up your children or grandchildren with ease? How about being able to safely climb onto a step stool to change a light bulb without needing assistance? What about being able to carry your groceries from the car into your home without having to take a break between trips? Exercise doesn't have to be a dirty word; we need only to understand its significance. I'm glad I finally do!

Tracking It

I remember talking with a parent at a soccer party about having recently started on my journey to better health. That parent told me about an app he was using and liked very much. The app he mentioned is MyFitnessPal. I downloaded it that very same day and have used it ever since. That was almost four years ago.

Using this tool has been a vital part of the turnaround in my health. It's very user-friendly and has been a "one-stop shop" for me. Not only have I been using it to track my food and water intake, but I can also make food and exercise notes there. It's on my phone, which is almost always with me; so, it's easily accessible, as well.

As I began to develop a routine for my daily eating habits, MyFitnessPal was much easier and more convenient for me to use than paper and pen. I discovered that I could use the app to plan for later in a particular day, or even for a future day.

Why was that important? Let's say that late in the morning, I had a craving for one of the brownies that a neighbor had sent as a treat for my family, and I wanted to eat it as an afternoon snack that day. I could search and enter "homemade brownie" in the app, and it would deduct the calories and nutrients from my daily allowance, showing me what I would have left for the day. That way, I could decide whether or not to have a brownie, as well as the portion of it.

It works the same way for future days. There have been times when I've made lunch plans with a friend for an upcoming week. Once we decided where we were going, I would go to that restaurant's website and look at the menu. I would choose a couple of options, and enter them both into MyFitnessPal. If I hadn't been getting quite enough protein in the week leading up to the lunch date, I would have the option that had more protein and delete the other choice from the app. This has worked very well for me.

I realized that I could use MyFitnessPal to import and save recipes from the internet that looked interesting. In addition, I could manually enter my own recipes by entering all of the ingredients and the total number of servings and save them in the app.

For instance, I could enter my recipe for homemade red beans and rice, estimating that it serves 12. When I'd choose a serving of that dish as a meal, the app would automatically divide the calories and nutrients by 12, providing an accurate account for the meal for each day that I would consume it.

If I eat the same meals regularly (for example: eggs, whole grain toast, and a banana for breakfast), I can copy and paste that meal from one day to the next. This makes it even more convenient to use.

Another great feature is being able to connect with others at your choosing, similarly to what many do on social media. It's nice to be able to see the progress that others are making, and they can see yours, again, if you so choose.

Using MyFitnessPal has helped keep me accountable to myself. Every five days, a message is displayed when I open the app telling me how many days I've logged in a row. In other words, it keeps a streak for me.

I like having the ability to take notes in the app. If there's an unplanned event, I can log it in Food Notes. If I set a personal record lifting weights or running, I can document it in Exercise Notes. I can also choose to record if I'm feeling sleepy or sluggish, if I've had a positive or negative reaction to something I've eaten, or just be aware if there is any type of pattern being developed, whether beneficial or detrimental.

Regarding exercise, if I want to add an exercise that isn't already in the app, I can create my own. This includes both strength (weights) and cardio exercises. It's nice to see if I'm progressing or regressing and why.

Please don't feel intimidated or discouraged if this sounds like so much information to absorb. Not everyone likes that much detail. I just wanted to share the ways that I've been enjoying using the app. It truly has been a tremendous tool to assist on my journey.

MyFitnessPal is certainly not the only app in existence to help people track progress in their health. However, it has been working extremely well for me personally. Maybe using a paper journal is easier for you. Perhaps, you prefer wearing a tracker on your wrist. Whether digital or manual, there is quite a variety of options available to provide assistance for those striving to improve their overall physical wellness. Whatever it is, finding what works best for YOU is clearly something important to do. That is key. This is what has aided me in achieving my health and fitness goals. I plan (in order) to succeed!

Eating and exercising with purpose was, and still is, a process for me; but, I am grateful to now understand this concept. We only have one body on this earth; it would be wise for us to take the best possible care of it. Would you agree? Regarding exercise, it can be a wonderful way to relieve stress. As far as food is concerned, my husband reminds me on occasion that food is fuel, providing the energy that our bodies need to function well. We are all trying to accomplish something in this life. Wouldn't it be nice if we were as healthy as possible to reach those goals?

Takeaway: Learning to consistently eat and exercise with purpose is essential in seeing positive changes in our health.

Action: Identify **one** change that you would be willing to make <u>this</u> <u>week</u> in the following areas:

(1) Food _____ Date: _____

(2) Exercise _____ Date: _____

Notes:

_____

_____

_____

Bridget McCray

3 ALTER YOUR THINKING

As I continued to read labels and make adjustments, I thought, "Man! It is so expensive to eat healthy!!" In being a stay-at-home mother for many years, the cost, in my mind, was surely something to be considered. As Dr. Walker and I spoke about this in conversation one day at the gym, she simply said, "Pay now, or pay later." Wow!! Those words still echo in my ears today. I had not looked at things from that perspective.

Count up the Cost

What did that mean? I strongly believe that, in a nut shell, it meant being worth it to make wiser choices on the front end, though they may seem more costly at the time, to avoid paying more than I realized I would have to pay on the back end. For example, if I chose to eat from the cheapest section of a fast food menu regularly, it wouldn't cost much money at that time. However, once I'd start having problems with my blood pressure because of the excessive amounts of sodium in those particular menu items, it would most likely cost me plenty:

> (1) *Money*: having to see a doctor and paying for prescription medication

(2) *Time*: waiting to see a doctor and waiting for a prescription to be filled
(3) *Physical wellness*: feeling less than my best
(4) *Emotional wellness*: feeling frustration knowing that I could have made smarter choices, but didn't

From that perspective, I'd have to ask myself if it was really worth it to buy cheap fast food.

Please understand that I'm not knocking fast food. Note that I mentioned the <u>cheapest</u> <u>section</u> of the menu. Many fast food restaurants now offer healthier options. As a busy mom with children who are very involved in school activities after school hours, sometimes there's no time to go home and eat before an event. When that happens in my family, we have our "go-to" places where we can enjoy the healthiest meals possible when we're on the go. The Lord knows what's involved in my schedule, but also provides wisdom to assist me as I desire to make better choices.

This also came to mind: I noticed that once I began to decrease my dairy intake, my face wasn't breaking out like it had been for so many years when I was consuming quite a bit of milk and other dairy products. This meant that I would not have to make frequent visits to see a dermatologist, nor use strong prescription medications that had terrible side effects, as I did when I was a teenager. I was no longer

buying practically every over-the-counter
or television-advertised acne product, only to use
them in part, because they didn't work well for me.

Let's not forget the small fortune I've spent on make-
up over the years, trying to cover up the acne
problem, but only exacerbating it. Dr. Walker helped
me to understand that a healthy body starts on the
inside. I would much prefer spending money on
foods that are better for my family and me, making us
healthier internally, instead of on external products
that only serve as bandages to temporarily cover up
problems, without addressing the root cause.

I strongly believe that if I had been making more
mindful eating choices years ago, I would not have
had to deal with acne, at least, not to the degree that I
did. Again, from that perspective, I would have to ask
myself if it was worth it to drink as much milk as I
wanted and consume as much sugar as I desired.

As I developed the habit of reading labels, which I
still do today, I felt a sense of empowerment. When I
go grocery shopping for my family, I have the
information I need to make the best all-around
decisions for the foods that we consume.

It's that Time of the Year!

What happens for loved ones' birthdays and
anniversaries? Thanksgiving? Christmas? We all know

these dates are coming every year, since they don't change. It can be a challenge to stay focused. Can't it? Honestly, who wants to practice mindful eating during these wonderful times of celebration?? I know I don't!

Taking one day at a time, I consciously began to plan ahead for these types of special occasions. Since I am pretty likely to splurge on those days, I intentionally make even wiser choices regarding diet and exercise on the days leading up to and the days following a holiday or special event.

The idea is the same for traveling to visit loved ones. For example, when my mom makes her fabulous gumbo or one of her delicious cakes while I'm visiting, believe me, I don't deny myself! However, I make sure to get at least 30 minutes of moderate-to-vigorous exercise most every day of my visit. I purposely stay on top of drinking enough water and eating my vegetables. Though it's a different environment, I don't have to give in to every craving that I may get. I could even invite loved ones to join me in mindfully making some wise choices. They may actually be receptive. We don't know if we don't ask. Right?

Next Gen

No one transforms his or her health overnight. It is, indeed, a process, especially as we get "younger". However, it is such an important step to take not only for us personally, but also for generations to follow: our children, their children, and so forth.

If we could give our children the tools they need to be their healthiest, in order to be able to accomplish their respective God-given plans on this earth, wouldn't we want to do that? It starts with us as parents; our children typically follow our example. We cannot honestly make demands that they eat healthier and get a sufficient amount of physical activity on a regular basis when they don't see us doing the same. I'm guessing that would sound hypocritical to them. (It certainly would to me.)

Whether we like it or not, we parents are all role models for our children, even in this area. We as mothers, in particular, are primarily the ones who buy the food that comes into our homes; we make the choices. If we don't buy junk food to have at home, our children can't eat it, because it isn't there to eat.

When I started to pay closer attention to my health and make different choices as it pertained to food, I understood that I could not expect for my children to change overnight. Why? Because this was not an overnight change for me, I could not insist that it be so for them. This would take time. I began the process of weaning my family from certain foods that had been like staples in our home.

For instance, we used to have a Sunday morning

tradition in our home: baked cinnamon rolls. They were from a can, not even homemade; but, oh my goodness, they were so very delicious! Hot, sweet, and gooey: YUM! It was a treat to which we all looked forward every week. Not only were the cinnamon rolls themselves sweet, but once they were baked, I covered them with the icing that came with them in the can. What did that mean? More processed sugar.

So that it would not be a shock to them, I told my family, our children in particular, that I was going to break the habit of having cinnamon rolls every Sunday. Instead of buying the rolls every week, I began to buy them less frequently. At first, it was every other week, then one week per month, then not at all. It's been approximately three years since we last had cinnamon rolls to eat in our home. In all honesty, we don't even miss them; no one asks for them. As I said, this is something that my family and I used to eat EVERY Sunday morning. Harmful habits can be broken if we're willing to put forth the effort to do so.

Weaning was a process, yet I found it interesting that there was very little resistance to it. It was the same thing with snacks. There were certain pre-packaged, baked snacks that I would buy for our children. The snacks were baked, so surely they were healthy. Or, were they? As I began to read the ingredients on the label, I thought, "Oh! No, no, no! We need to make a change!"

It was impressed upon my heart, I believe by God Himself, that I needed to start making snack bags of fruits and vegetables for my children; so, I did. I would put three different fruits and three different vegetables in a snack bag for each of them. I would use a combination of fruits that appealed to them: Mandarin orange slices, apple slices, grapes, strawberries, and blueberries. For raw vegetables, it wasn't quite as easy. I would put celery, cucumbers, and carrot slices in their bags, until one day, my son advised me that he really doesn't like celery. I told him that was fine and doubled up on his serving of cucumbers. He was still eating the vegetables, which was the objective. It didn't matter to me that they were not exactly the same as the ones my daughter was eating.

I explained that, for the time being, they would still be able to have their baked snacks, but I would be buying less of them and that they would need to eat their fruits and vegetables before having the baked snacks. It worked out really well. I showed my children how to clean and safely slice their fruits and vegetables, and they began doing so on their own. However, I had to set the tone for that. I am so thankful that I did and that they were still young enough to be able to make those adjustments without it being a major ordeal.

Let That Sink In

When trying to teach certain concepts to my children, I sometimes wonder if it's "sinking in". There was an instance a few years ago, in which there was a snow cone truck at my son's school after an event. He told me that he wanted to get one of those cold treats, but first read the nutrition label on the side of the truck. He saw that one snow cone contained 15 grams of sugar, which wasn't bad in his opinion. Though, when he looked more closely, he noticed that the size he'd originally planned to get had 30 grams of sugar. He was surprised by that and chose to get the smaller size. I was proud of him for making the wiser choice. It did sink in! (Notice I said " wiser" choice, not "perfect" choice.)

Recently, my daughter was given a box of candy as a prize for answering questions in her Sunday school class. She told me it was a candy she likes, but that she did read the nutrition label. She said, "Mom, it has 14 grams of sugar." After congratulating her for checking the label, I asked her to look again and tell me how many servings are in the box. Then, I explained that she has to multiply the 14g by the number of servings. When she did, she was shocked to find out that the box contained a whopping 126g of sugar, not to mention what the hard-to-read ingredients were! WOW!!

She then opted to only have a little bit and save the

rest for another time. Yes, I could have thrown the candy away, but I decided not to do so. Instead, I chose to delight in the fact that she had a sense of awareness for herself regarding what she was putting into her body. I was very proud of her. It did sink in!

As I alluded to earlier, whether we like it or not, the next generation IS watching us. They usually do what we do, as opposed to doing what we say to do, for our actions speak much more loudly than our words do. I truly desire to be an example worth following. Because I know better, I strive daily to do so, not only for my sake, but also for the sake of future generations.

Altering our thinking about what we can accomplish does take time, but it can be done. Maybe, you've tried every "quick fix" diet, pill, cream, or even surgery on the market, yet only saw temporary results. You could open a home gym with all of the exercise equipment and videos you've bought, all to no avail.

Could it be that you didn't think you could get healthier through something as simple as a balanced diet and regular exercise? Did your actions follow what you believed? Most likely, they did. Please don't ever forget that you CAN do all that you set your mind to doing. That's where real change starts.

Takeaway: Real change begins when we alter our thinking and align our steps with that new thought-process through practical application.

Action: What are three small, practical changes to which you would be willing to commit <u>this</u> <u>week</u>?

(1) _____ Date: _____

(2) _____ Date: _____

(3) _____ Date: _____

Notes:

_____

_____

_____

4 LEAVE BEHIND OLD HABITS

When I was growing up, my mom loved to cook and bake, and she was very good at it. (She still is!) She learned it from her mom, whom, I'm sure, learned it from hers, and so on. I especially looked forward to her homemade pralines and her cakes with homemade icing. Yum!!

As a child, I developed a love affair with sugar and with dairy, which continued into my adult life. I could eat sweet cereal for breakfast, lunch, and dinner, and I often did. Of course, I "had to" add more sugar to the already-sweetened cereal to get the taste just right. I almost always ate cereal with milk, as opposed to eating it dry, because it was more filling to me that way. So delicious!! Since I did not inherit my mom's love for cooking, this was a "win-win" for me…or, so I thought.

As a child, I got plenty of exercise and fresh air. At school, we would do sit-ups, chin-ups, push-ups, tumble sets, and other exercises to help build stamina and muscular strength every day in PE class. At recess, we would play kickball and tetherball, play on the monkey bars, and run freely in the schoolyard.

At home, I enjoyed roller skating, riding my bike, playing basketball and volleyball, and playing Frisbee with my friends. During most of my childhood, video games were not yet popular, so playing them was not a distraction from physical activity.

Subsequently, once I finished college, all of my regular physical exercise came to a screeching halt. As an accountant, my work did not require much movement. My life had become very sedentary. Though I'd occasionally walk a few flights of stairs at work, or power walk in the downtown area in which I worked at the time, it was just that: occasional.

I had always been proportionate in my build (bust, waist, and hips), so I'd never felt a need to make any changes. It had not occurred to me that the eating habits established in my earlier years could have been contributors to the excruciating migraines and to the severe acne that I experienced then. In addition, I did not realize that my then-sedentary lifestyle as an adult was also a factor, as I continued to deal with the migraines and the acne for decades more, roughly 35 years in total.

When my husband and I married almost 19 years ago, I still had these eating habits. My mom-in-law loved me to pieces (and still does), but surely did pray for me and for her son in this area. Why for her son? It is because she knew that I would be the one primarily shopping for and preparing meals in our home. She was concerned for my health, as well as for my husband's. Based on suggestions she'd made and based on observing her lifestyle, I'd made a few changes over the years, but they were not significant enough to see the results I didn't fully understand at the time that I needed to see.

Dare I forget to mention water? Unless it was to be used for cleaning something external (my body, dishes, clothes, etc.), I was not interested. Water was something that I rarely drank growing up, nor did I drink it as an adult for a long time. My idea of drinking water was having the juice from lemons squeezed into it and with lots of sugar; or adding sugar to already-sweetened tea; or guzzling a soda. They all contained water. Right? That was my logic at the time. I'd never seriously considered that drinking plain water would help to clean my body on the inside, not just on the outside.

I made a conscious effort to be intentional about establishing this new habit. I'd come to realize that it was very necessary for my physical well-being. I began putting a bottle of water next to the bed at night, so that I could start drinking it almost immediately after waking up. This meant that I could no longer use the excuse that I would have to go "all the way" to the kitchen to get it.

I would also take at least one bottle of water with me

in the car. I could drink it on the way home from picking up my children from school, on the way to an appointment, or while sitting at one of my children's events. It was the change in thinking about water that has allowed me to get to the place where I drink, at minimum, half my body weight in ounces of water just about every day. This took time, but my effort did pay off. I would never in a million years have imagined I would ever consume that much plain water…and, regularly!

Convenience Has a Price

I'd gotten the hang of reading labels, which was a giant step in the right direction. Now, it was time for me to move to the next level: doing more shopping in the perimeter of the grocery store. Why? It's because that's typically where the fresh produce is located, with fresh meats, poultry, and seafood not far away. The middle aisles generally contain more pre-packaged foods, many of which contain an abundance of additives and preservatives to give them shelf "life".

This seemed daunting at first. Let's face it: Life is busy! I have never really enjoyed cooking, so it would be super-convenient to just pick up a few family-sized, pre-packaged chicken dinners, seafood dinners, or pizzas. (Maybe, it was just me.) In roughly 30 minutes, my family and I could have a full meal without my having to be in the kitchen for much time.

Yet, convenience has a price. The more I read the
nutrition labels, the more I was amazed at the
amounts of sodium in some of those products, not to
mention several ingredients that I could hardly even
pronounce, much less knew what they were. I knew
that these could not be options for us, at least, not on
a regular basis. Nevertheless, I chose to approach
this with the same attitude discussed previously: one
choice at a time, one day at a time. Putting this basic
principle into practice has been extremely beneficial.

All or Nothing?

In my personal experience, getting healthy is not "all
or nothing". It is a gradual shift, breaking old,
harmful habits and establishing new, smarter habits.
Smarter habits, not perfect habits. I have learned that
trying to be perfect on this journey, or on any other,
can cause all sorts of frustration, which can lead to
physical problems (for me, headaches and nose
bleeds) and is counterproductive to pursuing good
health. No, thanks! I don't ever intend to travel that
road again.

I know the things that my family likes to eat.
Thankfully, my husband is not picky with food; he
"goes with the flow," which is a HUGE blessing.
Though I don't really enjoy cooking, I can cook, and
I do anyway, because it's a smarter choice for my

family. I encourage my children to add the things they would like to eat each week to the grocery app on my phone. This helps them to have a small part in the planning process. Hopefully, it will aid in preparing them to be adults who make responsible choices when planning meals and shopping for themselves, and someday, for their families.

I do my best to plan our meals every week. That way, I'm not having to make multiple trips to the grocery store, which almost always results in spending more than what was necessary. Everything goes on the list on my phone as we see that we need something. This keeps me from having to make a last-minute list, and possibly, from forgetting an item or two.

Do I do well with this every single week? Of course, I don't. Sometimes, I'm multi-tasking when we run out of something and don't remember to put it on the grocery list. Occasionally, when I buy produce, it ends up spoiling because of unplanned events that popped up during a particular week. Then, I have to make an extra trip to the store. Life happens to all of us, but I will say that having a plan in place has been quite useful and effective.

I also try never to go grocery shopping when I'm hungry. The times that I've done so haven't been pretty. My eyes wander, and I feel tempted to start putting things into the basket that I ordinarily would not and know that I should not. Strictly for the sake of convenience, I like to go right after I finish working out. To keep myself from making dumb decisions at the store, I make sure to drink enough water prior to going, which helps me feel full until I can eat. I want to do my best to set my family and me up for success.

Leaving behind old habits that hinder us is not an easy task, yet it is not unattainable. You used to eat a pint of your favorite ice cream every evening before bed in an effort to wind down. You used to eat almost the whole basket of breadsticks or chips brought to your table as you waited for the entrée you ordered at your favorite restaurant. You used to drink five sodas a day. You used to eat hot, delicious cinnamon rolls dripping with icing every week with your family. Can you identify with any of these? It may seem insurmountable to leave old, hindering habits behind, but it can be done…one choice at a time.

Takeaway: Old habits that cause harm can be broken with effort and consistency; new, helpful habits are established the same way.

Action: Record one harmful habit to which you would be willing to commit to work toward breaking this month and one wise habit that you plan to establish this month.

(1) I will actively start the process of breaking the

harmful habit of _____ on

_____.

(2) I will consciously begin to practice the wise habit

of _____ on

_____.

Notes:

_____

_____

_____

5 TEAM UP

Along my journey to physical wellness, I have been blessed with connections to some amazing people. Once I realized that I had to get serious about my health, I didn't know exactly what to do day-to-day. My mom-in-law was wonderful, as far as general ideas and suggestions for making improvements to my health. Dr. Walker was able to help me to go to the next level by providing even more practical ideas pertaining to my specific goals regarding both food and fitness.

I will say that I had to forget about being in my comfort zone, especially once I became a member of a gym. That's something I'd never before done, and on top of that, I didn't know a soul there. Oh my! I felt very uneasy at first.

It was easy to use a treadmill, a stair climber, or an elliptical. Yet, when it came to lifting weights, I was clueless. Like many others I've met, I had the misconception that if I started lifting weights, I would get bulky and look like a man. Oh, and the machines with weights, the ones with pictures on them that show you what to do: yep; I was still clueless, until…

Goodbye, Noise!

I was able to become a part of a small group of people that trained together every day. Before my husband joined the gym where I was a member, he encouraged me to observe, noticing who looked like he or she knew what to do. He could have trained me himself, since he's a former All-Star athlete, but his schedule did not allow it. Hiring a personal trainer was not an option at the time. There was a very kind gentleman, who showed the rest of us how the equipment worked and what proper form should look like.

Before I could be a part of that group, guess what I had to do? I had to get the noise out of my head, the noise that said, "You don't know what you're doing. Those folks don't want to be bothered with you. They're going to laugh at you." Blah, blah, blah! I had to decide that if I wanted to see something different in my health, I was going to have to be willing to do something different. I'm so glad I did!

From time to time, I would switch back and forth between working out on the weight floor and attending group fitness classes. Both were most definitely out of my comfort zone, because I grew up being pretty apprehensive about introducing myself to people. If a person didn't approach me first, we most likely would not have ever met. I wasn't being a snob; I simply lacked confidence.

Learning to team up with others has been an unexpectedly wonderful part of my journey. I've been at the same gym for almost five years now: for the first three, as a member, then as a certified group fitness instructor. I have the phone numbers of many people there and quite a few of us are connected on social media. There are a few with whom I have been blessed to develop deeper relationships, but those relationships began with similar goals regarding our health and fitness.

There have been times when I've seen one of the regulars and could tell that his or her countenance was not normal. As I would feel led to do so, I would ask if all is well with him or her and if I could pray with or for him or her. I've been blessed to also experience that shoe being on the other foot a time or two over the years. When you have a day that you feel heavy-hearted, and someone approaches you with sincerity, because he or she cares about you as a human being, and in an environment often stereotyped as a "meat market", it is absolutely priceless.

I have had many a day when I haven't felt like going, but went anyway. Once I arrive and see so many people working hard to improve themselves, I am motivated and thankful. Seeing them challenges me to want to do my best, as well. If I were to workout at home, I know myself well enough to know that I just wouldn't push as hard.

There are times when I cannot get to the gym. As I've said previously, life happens. However, I do my best to plan my schedule to include time for me to invest 20, 30, or 60 minutes in my health through exercise five days a week, at minimum. It is amazing to be able to do so alongside of others who are striving for something similar.

Teaming up with at least one like-minded person is a wonderful thing. Having at least one person, with whom you can share the joys and the setbacks of your journey to better health is encouraging. Having someone who understands where you are and what you're trying to accomplish, who cheers for you in the victories and cries with you during the difficult days, and all without judgment, is simply invaluable. You also get to be the person with whom someone else can share joys and setbacks. It's mutual, a partnership of sorts. I call this a "win-win".

Those closest to us, our family members and friends, may not necessarily have any interest in how much we were able to lift or push, or in how flexible we've become, and that's okay. This makes getting connected with those who have similar goals that much more important. Whether or not we want to admit it, we all need support from time to time. No man is an island, as the saying goes.

Takeaway: Partnering with at least one person, who has similar goals, can make the journey very effective and fulfilling.

Action: List three people you will commit to asking about being actively involved in your wellness journey.

(1) _____ Date completed: _____

(2) _____ Date completed: _____

(3) _____ Date completed: _____

Notes:

_____

_____

_____

6 **H**AVE FAITH

I had been planning often and was seeing success. Well, what happens when something comes up that is <u>unplanned</u>? Your child's after-school game lasts an hour longer than scheduled, and you haven't eaten yet. Without planning, you may be inclined to drive to the nearest fast food restaurant and get the least healthy item on the menu. How could one combat the temptation to do that?

I normally keep a snack in my purse just in case I'm inadvertently gone longer than I intended to be. It may be a protein bar or a small package of nuts or granola, just something to hold me over until I can eat a regular meal. I definitely keep a bottle of water handy, as well, when I'm driving from one place to the next.

When my husband spontaneously asks if I'd like to go to lunch or to dinner, I'm going. Period. That being said, what about if doing so would cause me to exceed my allotted amount of calories or sodium? Would I have sabotaged my progress?

From time to time, I'll hear someone at the gym talk about looking forward to a "cheat" meal. What is that anyway? It basically refers to a meal that is no longer part of a person's regular diet, yet the person really enjoys it, even though it may not be the healthiest option.

I used to say the same thing, until I learned to see it differently. I began to refer to that special meal as a "treat" meal. I work hard at tracking my food daily. I drink half my body weight in ounces of water just about every day. I exercise at least five days a week. Once I have a treat meal, which may be twice a month, if that, I've been doing this long enough to be able to go back to my usual diet without any issues. It took time to get to that place; it did not happen overnight.

In my journey, I've experienced that one bad day does not negate my progress. My husband would remind me to think of it like the stock market, looking at trends, not day-to-day numbers. Adopting this particular attitude has taken away lots of stress. I stopped beating myself up when I didn't have a perfect day. Who needs that added pressure?? I know I didn't.

So…what do you do when your co-worker unexpectedly brings your favorite donuts to work, and you didn't have a chance to eat breakfast before leaving home? What about when your neighbor sends hot, freshly baked bread, and it's the kind that you really like? Oh, and how about those fabulous cookies only sold in certain seasons by the cutest little ladies, to whom you dare not say "no"?

I'm guessing you might succumb to temptation in at least one of these scenarios. I certainly have! (Did my husband really have to buy **three** boxes of those cookies??) After your splurge, does that mean you should "throw in the towel" for the rest of the day? It doesn't have to be that way.

When I make a less than stellar choice for a meal or a snack, I decide to do better for the next meal. I refuse to allow myself to take the "I've already blown it, so I may as well go all the way" attitude. I would be setting myself up for certain failure, and I will not allow that to be an option.

More Than One Measure of Progress

From roughly May 2014 to September 2014, I lost 20 pounds and 10 inches in total, dropping four dress sizes. Weight loss was never my goal, but it did happen as a result of consistency in diet and exercise. In addition, I'm not taking any prescription medications and am glad about it.

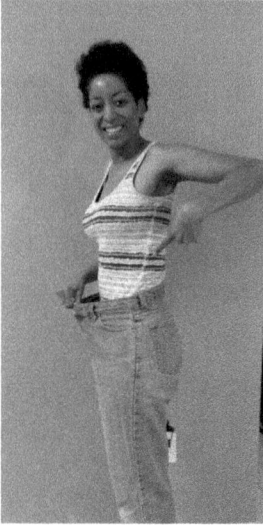

The process took longer for my skin…almost a year. It's the clearest that it's been in a long time. Though I may have an occasional flare up, that is much different than dealing with on-going acne. I did see a wonderful dermatologist early on, not just to take a food allergy test, but also because the scarring on my face was so bad from the acne, I wanted something to help fade them as rapidly as possible.

Admittedly, using a prescribed fade cream was a "quick fix" then. Yet, my intention was not to use it long-term. I thought that if I could continue to improve my eating and exercise habits, my skin would no longer break out, thus eliminating the need for fade cream in the future. I was right; that's exactly what happened.

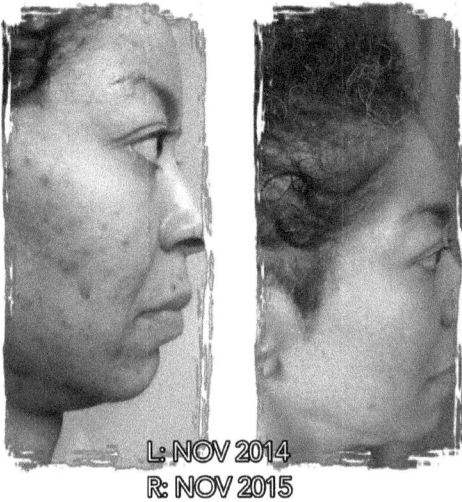

L: NOV 2014
R: NOV 2015

In our society, we are so conditioned to look at the scale to determine whether or not we're making progress physically. Seeing those numbers can be quite an emotional roller coaster, especially if one does it every day.

As you establish new habits, what if you notice that:

- You're sleeping better at night

- You have more energy

- The special jeans, in which you could once only barely breathe, now fit very well

- Your complexion is more evenly toned

- Your hair is softer and shinier

- You no longer hear creaking sounds when walking

- You can walk more than 15 feet without having to rest

- You've become flexible enough to reach your toes

Don't those things count? Sure, they do! The reading on the scale may not change much, but don't forget that it does not tell the whole story. Also, as we get stronger, our body composition begins to change; muscle occupies much less space than fat does. We should consider looking at the big picture; otherwise, discouragement will be headed our way. Slow progress is still progress. The point is to establish smart habits that will yield sustainable, long-lasting results.

In the beginning, I had this notion that the journey to better health and fitness had to be "all or nothing." There was little room for error in my mind at the time. I am so grateful to be free of that thinking. If I haven't learned anything else, I've discovered that consistency is key. I slowly began to appreciate the progress I was making, because I was no longer seeking perfection. As my husband would say: "Enjoy the wins along the way."

Are You Ready?

We all have to start somewhere. Whatever your first step may look like, the idea is to take it. Making the decision to do so is often the hardest part, yet it is not at all impossible. Your first move may not look the same as mine did. My aim in sharing in this book about what I've done to improve my physical well-being is to encourage and motivate people to simply get started.

So…you're willing to cast aside fears, past failures, and preconceived notions, and just "jump in". Congratulations! Now, what does that look like for YOU? Maybe, it means getting an extra half-hour of sleep. Perhaps, it means adding one day of intentional exercise per week. What about substituting one bottle of water for a soda that you would normally drink? Could it be eating a raw salad containing dark leafy greens with your lunch or dinner and without drowning it in dressing?

The road to better health is not as difficult as one may perceive it to be, but it does require regular, continued effort. As my husband would say, "Chopping down a tree takes consistency in hitting the same spot."

My heart's desire was to be transparent in this book about both the joys and the challenges I have experienced on my journey to wellness. Here is an acronym, H.E.A.L.T.H., that you may find to be a practical tool as you embark upon your own personal journey:

H - **H**ave a plan with small, attainable goals.

E - **E**at and exercise with purpose.

A - **A**lter your thinking about what you can accomplish.

L - **L**eave behind old habits that hinder you.

T - **T**eam up with at least one like-minded person.

H - **H**ave faith that you can achieve what you desire.

I have used each of these as chapter titles, as well, in an effort to reinforce some simple ideas that you, the reader, might find useful in making a lifestyle change.

Have faith that you can achieve what you set out to do. Whenever there was a time I thought I couldn't do something, I was right. I would actually talk myself out things before I even tried. That was "stinking thinking"! Each one of us has a purpose on this earth. We can reach our dreams. My faith is in the Creator of the heavens and the earth. I know that through His Son, Jesus Christ, I can, indeed, do all things. It is through Him that I have the strength to continue when I feel like quitting, or when I feel like giving in to the temptations that come. With faith and hard work, we can do great things! Without works, our faith is dead.

The Wrap-Up

Before I started paying attention to my health, I naively thought that everything was fine solely based on the fact that I was considered shapely. Little did I know that this was no guarantee of good health.

It was tough to be of service to my family and others, to work, or to do much of anything when I wasn't feeling well. It was an incredible challenge to care for my children, who were then toddlers, when I used to have migraines. There was little-to-nothing I could do for them during those times of indescribably intense pain. I do not miss having those at all!!

And, the acne…though it did not physically hurt for the most part, it was hard looking into the mirror every day and seeing my skin in that awful condition for so long. It was an emotional drain, and I felt a sense of hopelessness, like I was literally doomed to have ugly, bumpy, scarred skin for life.

Never in my wildest dreams would I have imagined that working through a blood pressure problem, which had suddenly manifested in my life, would become a source of encouragement and motivation for others.

I will tell no lie; there have been struggles along the way. There have been days when I haven't wanted to eat the things I know that I should. There have been

days when I have not felt like going to the gym. My journey has been far from perfect. Yet, I have learned how to navigate those days, one choice at a time.

Regardless of the struggles, I am truly grateful that whether physical (feeling tired) or mental (not feeling confident that I could push or lift a certain amount of weight), they have helped me to grow, and not only in reference to my physical health. I am definitely mentally stronger as a result of being on this journey.

For years, I'd prayed to the Lord to take away the migraines and the acne. For years, it felt as if my prayers had fallen on deaf ears. Then one day, these words came to mind: "I will always do My part. Now, what are YOU going to do? Faith without works is dead." It had finally clicked! I understood! I was expecting God to work a miracle, as if I weren't responsible to do anything at all. I had faith that He would help, but I initially had no works as evidence of that faith. Thus, I'd only seen little change back then.

He helped me, indeed. Every step of the way, He was with me, and He still is. How thankful I am for the breath He allows to flow through my body, even when I'm not "in the mood" to make wise decisions. He is with me then, too. What a merciful God!

When others questioned why I chose to work so hard to improve my health through changes to my lifestyle, saying, "You've got to die of something", then proceed to purposely tempt me with food or try to dissuade me from exercise; when there was snickering about how (they felt) I was getting too skinny; my God was with me. He always is.

Though there were certain things I wanted to accomplish in reference to my health, developing a healthy lifestyle was merely a discipline, something I needed to do in order to help me fulfill His design for my life and do so without hindrance. Experiencing physical wellness has been a goal within a much bigger plan for me.

I hope that my story has been a source of inspiration and motivation for you. As a result of personally experiencing what it's like to change how I think about food and exercise, I have been able to document many of those things here, in this book, in order to be able to encourage others.

If I can change my lifestyle for the better, so can you. It starts with one choice. You are worth it. What is the alternative? A commitment to this lifestyle is not impossible, but it does take effort. Is the cost of doing nothing truly worth it?

There's no time like the present. Please don't wait until tomorrow to start taking care of yourself, for it is not promised. You were created to accomplish great things. Wouldn't it be wonderful to be able to do them to the fullest without having to worry about your health?

May the Lord bless you as you embark upon the journey to a healthier YOU. You <u>can</u> do it! Remember, it's not rocket science.

Takeaway: Having faith as you put the concept of H.E.A.L.T.H. into practice can help as you begin the journey to a healthier you.

Action: Complete the Self-Evaluation in the Worksheet section of the book.

Notes:

_____

_____

_____

WORKSHEETS

Bridget McCray

SELF-EVALUATION WORKSHEET
(Part 1 of 3)

(1) WHY would you like to improve your health? (for your family; to be able to travel, start a business, change careers, fulfill a lifelong dream; etc.)

_____

_____

_____

(2) Do you feel you are worth the investment of time and effort? _____

(3) What are some potential obstacles that you foresee as you seek to get healthier?

_____   _____

_____   _____

_____   _____

(4) What are some ideas to help overcome those possible stumbling blocks?

_____   _____

_____   _____

SELF-EVALUATION WORKSHEET
(Part 2 of 3)

After reviewing the action steps at the end of each chapter:

(5) Did you follow-through with each one to which you committed? _____

(a) If so, how did it feel?

_____

(b) If not, why not?

_____

(6) Which action step(s) is (are) going well for you, and how?

_____

_____

(7) Which action step(s) is (are) not working as well, and why?

_____

_____

SELF-EVALUATION WORKSHEET
(Part 3 of 3)

(8) What adjustments are you willing to make over the next six months in order to invest in YOUR overall wellness?

_____   _____

_____   _____

_____   _____

_____   _____

_____   _____

Date completed: _____

PERSONAL PROGRESS TRACKING WORKSHEET

Inspired Me	Date	Date	Determined Me	Date	Consistent Me	Date	Improve Me
	Week 1	Week 2	Change	Week 3	Change	Week 4	Change
Weight*							
Waist**							
Bust**							
Lower Abs**							
Hips**							
Thigh-L**							
Thigh-R**							
Upper Arm-L**							
Upper Arm-R**							

Here's to becoming a HEALTHier you!

* In pounds
** In inches

ACCOMPLISHMENTS

(1) _____

Date: _____

(2) _____

Date: _____

(3) _____

Date: _____

(4) _____

Date: _____

(5) _____

Date: _____

(6) _____

Date: _____

(7) _____

Date: _____

(8) _____

Date: _____

Bridget McCray

DISCLAIMER

I am not affiliated with MyFitnessPal and/or Under Armour, Inc. MyFitnessPal and Under Armour do not promote, support, and/or approve the material and contents of this book in any form.

Front cover photo
by JESHOOTS.COM on Unsplash

For speaking engagements and/or social media
information, please visit www.bridgetmccray.com.